Ultimate Atkins Diet Quick Start Tool Kit!

I0419812

Atkins Diet

A Complete Low Carb Recipe Book To Lose Weight And Feel Great With Proven Scientific Techniques For Rapid Fat Loss!

Sarah Brooks

Legal Notice

Disclaimer Notice

Table Of Contents

Introduction

Chapter 1 – Why Atkins Diet?

Chapter 2 – Weight Loss And Atkins Diet

Chapter 3 – The 4 Phases Of Atkins Diet

Chapter 4 - 10 Amazing Atkins Diet Recipes

Chapter 5 – Grocery Shopping Tips For Atkins

Chapter 6 – How To Go Out To Eat On The Atkins Diet

Chapter 7 - Top Foods To Eat And Foods To Avoid

Chapter 8 - Health Benefits Of The Atkins Diet

Chapter 9 – Avoiding Crucial Mistakes

Chapter 10 - Staying Motivated

Conclusion

Preview Of: "Low Carb Diet:Low Carb Diet Plan For Fat Loss For Life! Fast Acting Low Carb Diet To Lose Weight As Soon As Tomorrow!"

Free Bonus Offer

Introduction

I want to thank you and congratulate you for purchasing the book, *Ultimate Atkins Diet Quick Start Tool Kit! Atkins Diet: A Complete Low Carb Recipe Book To Lose Weight And Feel Great With Proven Scientific Techniques For Rapid Fat Loss!*

This "Atkins Diet" book contains proven steps and strategies on how to lose weight and keep the desired weight forever. Most diets are only good in keeping off the excess weight for a short time. The moment hunger and the cravings set in, weight creeps back with a vengeance. However, Atkins diet is so effective that you can live off it for the rest of your life.

Detailed in this book are ways on how to greatly benefit from this diet and avoid regaining the lost weight. Included also are measures to undertake should your weight loss endeavors fall off course.

The next step is to read this book, follow the steps outlined and share the knowledge contained in it with friends, families and college.

Enjoy!

Thanks again for purchasing this book, I hope you enjoy it!

Chapter 1 – Why Atkins Diet?

It has been a common knowledge among experts in the past that the way to treat obesity is to maintain a balance between caloric intake and expenditure. Simply put, in order for a person to lose weight, one must consume less calories than their energy requirement for the day. Doctors who were assisting obese people in their weight loss efforts in the past have prescribed caloric limitations through behavioral restraint.

During early 1950's, experiments and studies by various experts have revealed a hurdle to this concept. While it is true that weight loss can be initiated by limiting the amount of caloric intake compared to what the body actually uses up, scientists have found out that doing so causes the body's metabolic rate to drop. The requirement for energy by the body drops due to a decrease in the activity in each tissue of the body resulting in a lower energy requirement to operate. Experts have further observed that obese people living off a limited amount of calories equal to that of a lean exhibited no fat loss over time as their body's metabolism tends to dip.

An inspiration and a success story

In 1958, an article written by Alfred A. Pennington entitled "Weight Reduction" about research papers conducted on weight loss and caloric restriction and published on The Journal of the American Medical Association inspired Robert Atkins to use the study to resolve his own weight-related problems.

Atkins achieved a successful weight reduction from his weight of 100 kg (224 pounds) by following a restrictive diet almost devoid of starch and sugar (as indicated in the study of Pennington) and found that the effect was instant and lasting. This prompted him to share his findings and began advertising its effects on patients. Concordantly, an article investigating Pennington's research entitled "A New Concept in the Treatment of Obesity" published in the Journal of the American Medical Association by Edgar S. Gordon, Marshall Goldberg and Grace J. Chosy supported the advocacy of eliminating sugar and starch from the diet and supplementing the body's caloric requirements through protein and fat. The diet was soon popularized through a series of books by Atkins which was initially published in 1972. The diet has since underwent many modifications and has advanced to be one of the widely used weight-loss diet that effectively addresses the root of weight-loss issues in obese persons.

Pervasiveness and Popularity

The popularity of Atkins diet had its peak and had its abrupt dip during 2003-2004. One in 11 North American adults found that the carbohydrate-restrictive diet was so effective they lived-out on it causing a significant decrease in carbohydrate-rich foods and products like rice and pasta and striking a heavy blow on Krispy Kreme sales. The dip, however, on the prevalence of this diet was caused by the death of Dr. Atkins on 2003 after an accident.

Reason for Preference

Any weight loss diet will fall into this demise if left unchecked—your body will detect your efforts to starve it and will go into a state in which the caloric expenditure is reduced while fat storage is maximized. Because of this, a person can go on limiting his caloric intake and still gain weight while suffering the physiological and the emotional discomforts of the process.

Experts believe that the reason for this is the consumption of carbohydrates as a source of calories. Because carbohydrates can easily be converted into readily absorbed and utilized form, the body tends to resort to using it as a primary energy source. Consequently, under a low carbohydrate condition, our body resorts to a low metabolic state. Studies have vaguely revealed that the reason for this is not necessarily caloric deficit as any deficit is accounted for by the body's caloric reserves but rather the inability of the body to effectively mobilize the adipose tissues to provide for the deficit in the energy supply.

Atkins Diet is particularly effective against this as its main attribute is low consumption of carbohydrates. This ensures that blood sugar is constantly kept at a minimum level therefore eliminating the necessity for the body to produce insulin. Under low levels of sugar and insulin, the body enters a state called *ketosis*. Experts agree that ketosis is the best condition a body could be to maximize mobility of and minimize the oxidation of adipose tissues.

Other reasons to choose Atkins diet over other diets:

- **More fats are mobilized as energy source.** A recent study conducted by Stanford University involving 311 obese premenopausal women comparing four calorie restrictive diet (Atkins, Zone, Eat More, Weigh Less, and LEARN reveal that Atkins dieters shed more pounds than those who were under the three other diet programs. The research further reveals that Atkins dieters have better cardiovascular conditions as they exhibit improved blood pressure and healthy serum levels of HDL cholesterol and triglycerides. One of the researchers remarked that the answer may lie on the *drastic reduction of dietary carbohydrates*—a primary attribute of the Atkins diet.
- **Dieters do not experience hunger.** Unlike most diets which focuses on caloric restriction regardless of the caloric source (be it protein, fats or carbohydrate) and rely on caloric intake measurement, Atkins diet, by essence, is not restrictive and dieters do not face the challenge of hunger of depravity in achieving their weight loss goals. The only restriction Atkins imposes is that of carbohydrates. Carbohydrates are chains of sugar molecules which are easily digested and utilized by the body for energy. Carbohydrates also serve as a deterrent in achieving ketosis—the primary mechanism of weight loss in Atkins diet.
- **Maintaining a desired weight is easier.** Initially, the effects of almost all forms of diets available today are similar. It affords you a rapid decrease in weight (either true weight or excess water weight) but as soon as the physiological and psychological discomforts associated with starvation and prolonged caloric restrictions sets in, and the moment a dieter indulges in food, all the lost weight returns as a rebound effect. The secret lies in what experts discovered in 1994—a hormone they now call the "starvation hormone" (erroneously referred by some as the "obesity" hormone) called *leptin*. Leptin is a hormone produced in the fat cells believed to regulate weight (or keeps the body from

losing weight). When a person's body undergoes a rapid weight loss, the amount of leptin in the blood decreases consequently. This tells the brain that the body is experiencing a deficiency in its caloric supply. Shortly after this, the brain prompts the body to decrease its metabolism—a state in which the over-all energy expenditure of every cells in the body decrease—and instructs each cell to store excess energy as fat. Although Atkins dieters also experience a decrease in the amount of leptin in their blood, this is only temporary and may last from 10-30 days. During which the body adapts to ketosis. After which, the level of leptin normalizes and the discomforts associated with reduced serum levels of leptin goes away.

- **It does not deprive you of food or of energy.** In Atkins diet, you need not count your caloric intake. You are allowed to eat as much as you can as long as you follow a prescribed ratio between fat and protein and as long as you keep your carbohydrate level to a certain prescribed amount. During the initial phase of Atkins diet (and of ketosis), you might feel sluggish and a little short of energy but eventually, after your body has completely adapted to ketosis, your energy will be increased to such a level higher than when your body was dependent on glucose for energy. Unlike other diets which make you feel sluggish, Atkins diet makes you feel energized longer. This means you no longer force yourself to exercise but you are motivated to do so because you feel more alive.
- **The diet plan is healthy.** Various clinical studies and researches conducted in the past revealed that reducing the amount of carbohydrates in the diet greatly decreases a person's likelihood of contracting cardiovascular diseases by improving the serum levels of LDL cholesterol and triglycerides, normalizing the blood pressure and maintaining a healthy serum level of glucose. In addition, Atkins diet features a holistic nutritional approach as opposed to purely ketogenic diet programs.
- **Keeps insulin levels at safe levels.** Carbohydrate dependent diets are diets that favor the presence of large quantities of glucose in the blood specially those

which is composed of processed carbohydrates. Increase and frequent spike in blood glucose levels prompts the body to release insulin to neutralize the sugar. However, at prolonged exposure, the cells of the body becomes desensitized to the effect of the insulin and that higher levels of insulin are required to bring about its normal effect in each cell. This condition is more commonly referred to in the medical world as insulin resistance. Insulin resistance is a risk factor for developing diabetes and cardiovascular diseases. Atkins diet is low in sugar and carbohydrates. As a matter of fact, the process takes your body from a state of being fully depended on carbohydrates (and sugar) for energy to a state where it is an efficient user of stored energy. Atkins diet does cause an increase in insulin levels in the blood, prevents the diseases associated with insulin resistance and is a viable lifestyle alternative more than just a dietary regimen.

Chapter 2 – Weight Loss And Atkins Diet

Aside from the pesky excess water weight (that dieters often mistake to be a significant weight lost during the initial stages of a restrictive diet, excess weight can be attributed to the weight of stored fats (either as brown, white or visceral fat). When we speak about weight loss, we refer to the process of eliminating (or using up) as much fat as we can by converting them to usable forms though activities such as physical exercise or dieting.

The human body, however, has a resilient mechanism that does not favor the easy conversion of fat to energy, especially if there is an abundant supply of glucose in the blood—an energy source that the body favors. In the presence of blood glucose, the body responds by prompting the beta-cells of the pancreas to produce insulin which carries the glucose from the blood to every tissues in the body and be used for fuel. At low serum levels of glucose (hence at low serum levels of insulin), the body falls short of energy necessary to maintain its usual metabolic processes. In order to compensate for the depravity, the body enters a state which utilizes fat as an alternative energy source.

Ketosis

The state at which the body begins utilizing fat reserves as an energy source is called ketosis. In order to enter ketosis, blood glucose must be reduced to an amount less than 64.5 mg/dl or 3.58 mmol/liter. Atkins diet limits the daily consumption of carbohydrates to about 20 net grams. With this amount of dietary carbohydrate, Atkins diet effectively induces ketosis (and is categorized as a *ketogenic diet.)*

The small amount of carbohydrates included in an Atkins dieter is not enough to supply the blood with enough glucose to activate its insulin response. The amount of insulin in a dieter's blood allows its body to gauge the energy the body gets. With this few insulin, the body is informed of an insufficiency in the energy supply and triggers processes that enables it to utilize other sources of energy (i.e. adipose deposits and protein reserves).

During a state of hypoglycemia (or glucose deficiency in the bloodstream), the body responds by sending out growth hormones such as cortisol, growth hormones, epinephrine and glucagon to facilitate the release of stored glycogen from the liver and from the conversion of triacylglycerol (from adipose deposits) to fatty acids.

In order for the body to use fats (adipose tissues) for energy, growth hormones and epinephrine are released to convert triacylglycerol (fats) to fatty acids. These fatty acids are then oxidized in the liver and in the muscles to be converted to acetyl-CoA before it can be used by the cells for energy. Excess acetyl-CoA are converted by the liver to ketones where they are either transported to tissues to be converted back to acetyl-CoA for energy or filtered by the kidney and released via the excretory system as a waste product.

Atkins as a Lifestyle

When your weight increased to such a degree as you have now, your life has changed. You no longer play the games you once did, perform the activities you once did with ease, wear the same size of clothes to flatter your figure or have the same amount of confidence as you once had.

As frightening as it may appear to change a lifestyle, you might not notice (before now) that you have had underwent a lifestyle change. You only failed to notice it because the transition was gradual.

Atkins diet, without the actual intent to fright you, is more than just a diet. It is a lifestyle change that must be adapted throughout the remainder of your (long) life. If you are looking for a diet that would afford you an instant weight loss in a short duration of time, there are many in the market (including Atkins). If you are looking for a diet that would enable you shed a few pounds in a short period of time and allow you to gorge in to any food you want without gaining the weight afterwards, you are not looking for a diet—you are looking for a cheat code for life and frankly nothing such as that exists.

The usual diet of a typical American from birth to his present age is largely determined by the available food within his reach (usually provided by the food industry in his locale). This, however, does not guarantee that the diet and the type of food he was brought up with is the right kinds of food. Data from the President's Council on Fitness, Sports and Nutrition provides that the typical American diets exceeds the allowed intake levels of calories from added sugars, refined grains and sodium and includes less than recommended amounts of vegetables, fruits, oils and dairy products. Furthermore, experts, including Christopher J.L. Murray

Atkins diet is not an ideal temporary weight loss remedy that a dieter should be at for a couple of months or so or until he achieves his desired weight. Experts have long since understood that the body has an internal gauge that remembers a person's weight and prevents him from shedding pounds. With the right opportunity and resources, the body tends to recover the said weight. This explains why the body tends to lower its caloric expenditure following days of caloric deprivation. This also explains why a person readily recovers back the weight he just lost as soon as he stops the diet. This mechanism, which seems to be greatly regulated by the brain, is still poorly understood.

Atkins diet, however, is one (if not the best) of the ideal diets that could be adapted for life because it does not deprive a person of food. In fact, its foundations are laid down on the premise that a dieter must not be deprived of food. As soon as you grasp the entirety of the concept, you will realize why.

Eat more. Lose weight.

For years, experts have propagated the idea (which is true) that in order to lose weight, one must lessen the amount of food (calories) he takes in and expend more energy (through exercise). This is a fact and this is backed up by a hardcore scientific law, the first law of thermodynamics: energy is neither created nor destroyed. Thus, what you take in must be what is inside you; and in order to lessen what is inside you, you must reduce the energy you take in and increase the energy you use up. However, the revolutionary diet followed by almost 17 million people around the world known as Atkins diet, seems to defy this law because, in essence, it instructs to eat as much as you want to help you lose weight.

Proponents of Atkins have found an explanation for this. Excess ketones, a byproduct of processing fat used by cells to generate energy, is not stored as fat as opposed to excess blood sugar from carbohydrates. Instead, scientists have found out that excess ketones are removed from the body through urine. In essence, achieving ketosis through Atkins diet affords a person the chance of actually peeing off excess calories.

Another reason for this is that protein has been found out to reduce appetite. Atkins diet is particularly rich in protein which may explain that although dieters are allowed as much food as they want, they feel less hungry and are more satisfied and tend to eat less carbohydrate compared to dieters of other diet programs.

Chapter 3 – The 4 Phases Of Atkins Diet

The purpose of all carbohydrate restrictive diet is to attain *ketosis*. Only in this state can the body achieve a maximum efficiency in utilizing its fat reserves for energy. However, ketosis is not a body state that a person achieves in a couple of days or so after refraining from carbohydrate intake. A body so dependent to glucose, a quick source of energy, will not easily change to a fat-dependent one. Some individuals, in fact, have systems so resilient it appears to prevent ketosis in its desire to prompt the individual to ingest carbohydrates.

Experts have divided the phases involved in Atkins diet in order to prescribe a more specific diet composition for each phase and thus maximize the effect of the diet while eliminating potential discomforts associated with weight loss (particularly rapid ones).

- **Phase I – Induction Phase.** Of all the phases of Atkins diet, this is the most restrictive and the most crucial. During this stage, the body if *forced* to enter into ketosis. This is done by limiting the carbohydrate intake to as little as 20 grams per day with most of carbohydrates coming from vegetables such as tomatoes, asparagus, turnips, broccoli, spinach, pumpkin and cauliflower. Other foods that are allowed are some 54 vegetables (which will be covered in a separate chapter about foods to eat), meat, fish, shellfish, eggs, fowl and poultry (at 5-6 ounces every meal), hard and semi-soft cheeses (at 4 ounces), and fat sources such as olive oil, vegetable oils and butter. Caffeine and alcoholic beverages are not allowed during this phase as excess ketones are expected to be excreted through the kidneys. These substances are known to either add up to the burden of kidney or interfere altogether with achieving ketosis. Here are the steps to do induction correctly:

  - **Don't starve yourself.** An indicator that you are not doing Atkins right is the feeling of depravity and hunger. It is important that you indulge in your cravings for food. As much as possible, do not go more than 6 hours without eating. A typical Atkins eating pattern is three meals and 2 snacks a day. However, to maximize fat burning, one could adapt a 6 small meals a day taken at a three-hour interval.

- **Consume 20 grams of carbohydrates a day.** No ifs, no buts, and no exception. This is not a rule just made up by Dr. Atkins himself. If you consume more than the maximum carbohydrate required to enter ketosis, you might divert your system back to carbohydrate-based metabolism which will render all your past efforts to enter ketosis futile. The next time you tell yourself to *actually* limit your carbohydrate intake will take you to the first day of induction again. There are even instances where people's body become increasingly sensitive to carbohydrates and encourages a gush in insulin which could accelerate the deadly process of insulin-resistance in their systems.

- **Concentrate on protein.** You don't want your body to start burning off your muscles for energy instead of your adipose deposits which is typical during low-carbohydrate conditions. Ingesting more proteins would give your body the protein it needs without resorting to getting it from your muscles.

- **Eat fat.** Not only do fats add flavor to foods and make every eating experiences enjoyable, it is also a key factor in maintaining ketosis. If you are worried about the health hazards of high fat diet, you can safely opt for healthy fat sources. These unsaturated and polyunsaturated fat sources are not stored in the body as fat as opposed with other sources of fat. Furthermore, as stated in the previous chapters, as fats are broken down to ketones, excess ketones are flushed out of urine instead of being stored/restored as fats in the body.

- **Keep yourself well hydrated.** Ketones are known to acidify blood and increase the need for the body to balance out the blood pH. The body does this by increasing calcium intake in the intestines and calcium leaching in the bones. Because of this, Calcium excretion through the urine is increased. This adds burden to the kidneys and insufficient hydration favors the development of kidney stones. It is important that the urine is well diluted by ensuring enough hydration to prevent kidney-related problems associated with Atkins (and all other ketogenic) diets. The ideal water consumption is 8 8-ounce water a day.
- **Don't go easy on salt.** Salt may actually be helpful here as the initial weight lost during Atkins is water-weight. This is due to the decline in the amount of electrolytes in the blood. Include salt by adding salty broth, soy sauce and table salt in your diet.
- **Be wary of hidden carbs.** Look out for hidden carbohydrates in foods. They may not take the form of the usual white flour or sugar but they sure are part of the ingredients of the food. Among those are mayonnaise, flavorings, coffee, artificial sweeteners, spices, and even eggs. Be sure to count the number of carbohydrates in them properly while being cautious not to exceed the daily recommendation of 20 grams. The full list of foods and their hidden carbohydrates content will be dealt with in the succeeding chapters.
- **Go easy on sugar substitutes.** Although they are preferable compared to table sugar as they contain fewer calories, they still contain carbohydrate components and should be treated a carbohydrate source. An article published on 1987 in the journal "Hormone and Metabolic Research" revealed that the artificial sweetener acesulfame-K tends to cause the release of insulin just as glucose would.

Suggested usage quantity is no more than 3 packets per day.

- **Phase II – On Going Weight Loss.** The goal of this phase is to select the critical carbohydrate intake a person's body could tolerate. This is done by gradually introducing a small amount of carbohydrate in the diet by 5 grams a week. This phase usually continues until the dieter is within 4.5 kg of his desired weight. This is introduced by consuming nuts and seeds on the first week of the phase followed by a *carbohydrate ladder* (introduction of carbs in an increment of 5 grams per week) and berries (for antioxidants). Foods such as legumes, high-carb fruits and vegetables and whole grains are not continued on the final phase. The foods are included only in this phase.

- **Phase III – Pre-maintenance.** During this, the net carbohydrate intake is increased by a weekly increment of 10 grams. This time, the maximum amount of carbohydrate is determined upon which a dieter could include in his diet without actually gaining weight. Dieter is encouraged to take in liberal amounts of liquid during this phase.

- **Phase IV- Lifetime Maintenance.** This is the final phase of the Atkins' diet. The goal is to carry on the carbohydrate intake patterns acquired in the previous phases. Processed foods are discouraged and maintaining the carbohydrate diet is preferred. Whenever a person starts to gain weight, he is advised to return to the previous phase.

Chapter 4 - 10 Amazing Atkins Diet Recipes

No Carb Mushroom Omelet

Egg whites provide a great amount of protein, are easy to make and if done properly, can be very delicious! Here is a great low carb and low fat, high protein recipe:

Ingredients:

1 cup mushrooms (sliced)
1 cup of Spinach
1 cup Zucchini (grated)
1 tablespoon Paprika
12 egg whites
Salt
Pepper
1 teaspoon Fresh Oregano

Here's how:

1. Combine and process the ingredients in a blender excluding the mushrooms.
2. Heat a lightly greased pan with coconut oil.
3. Pour the mixture in the pan and cook it like omelet.
4. Add the mushrooms on top of the omelet and finish cooking.
5. Serve hot and enjoy.

Versa Pancakes

This dish is perfect either as a snack or as a breakfast.

Ingredients:

1 cup oats
1 teaspoon baking powder
1 cup unsweetened almond ilk
12 egg whites
Stevia (to taste) or any preferred artificial sweetener
2 teaspoons of cinnamon

1 cup Frozen Blueberries
1 cup Unsweetened Applesauce

Here's how:

1. Process egg whites, baking powder, oats, salt, almond milk and stevia in a food processor.
2. Add a quarter of the blueberries to the blended mixture.
3. Cook the mixture on a pan lightly greased with coconut oil.
4. Top the pancakes with applesauce, stevia, cinnamon and the remainder of blueberries.
5. Serve.

Omelet Sud-Ovest

Ingredients:

1-2 garlic cloves minced
1/3 cup spinach chopped
1/4 cup fat-free cottage cheese
2 tablespoon salsa (prefer the low-carb and no-sugar variants)
1/2 teaspoon chili powder
1 teaspoon coconut oil
1/3 cup green onion
1/3 cup mushrooms (chopped)
6 egg whites
Salt and pepper to taste

Here's how:

1. Pour the oil over the cooking pang and heat it over high settings.
2. Add in and sauté the onion, garlic and mushrooms until soft.
3. Set the mixture aside.
4. Oil the pan and pour in the egg whites.
5. Add in the mixture on top of the white eggs and cook (while the pan is covered).
6. Flip over the omelet and cook for another minute or two.
7. Remove the omelet from the heat and top it with spinach, cheese and salsa.
8. Fold the omelet and serve.

No Fry Seafood Omelet

This recipe is perfect for those who are hesitant about the amounts of fat included in the diet. It contains less carbs and fats than most omelets and is packed with appetite-zapping proteins.

2 tablespoon cottage cheese (melted; preferably fat free)
1/2 teaspoon tarragon
100 grams shrimp (cooked; preferably fresh)
Salt and pepper to taste
4 egg whites
1 teaspoon coconut oil

Here's how:

1. Whisk the tarragon, cottage cheese and eggs together in a medium sized food bowl.
2. Heat the oven to 375.
3. Heat and grease a skillet with coconut oil.
4. Pour the mixture prepared in 1 to the pan and add the shrimp on top.
5. Place the skillet on the oven and let it bake for 5-7 minutes.
6. Take the omelet out of the oven and fold in half.

All-Protein Pancake

We absolutely love this recipe and would have it almost daily until just a few weeks before our competition. It takes no time to make and it feels like a real treat!
Ingredients:

1/2 scoop of whey protein isolate powder
1/4 teaspoon baking powder
2 tablespoon ground flaxseed
4 egg whites
1 teaspoon coconut oil

Here's how:

1. Blend the ingredients in a food processor.
2. Meanwhile, heat a medium sized cooking pan and lightly grease it with coconut oil.

3. Pour half of the mixture into the pan and cover.
4. Let it cook for 4-5 minutes.
5. Flip the pancake over and cook the other side for a minute or so.
6. You can top it with a quarter of cinnamon with 3 packets of Stevia.

Bunless Seafood Burgers

This seafood based burgers require no bun and are carb free. It allows you to enjoy the taste without the guilt.

Ingredients:

200g cooked shrimp
2 large Portobello mushroom caps
1 leek, finely chopped
2 egg whites
1 clove garlic, crushed
1/2 teaspoon onion powder
1 tablespoon Worcestershire sauce
2 tablespoon ground flax seeds
2 tablespoon fat free low sodium cottage cheese salt and pepper (to taste)

Here's how:

1. Heat the oven to 450. Meanwhile, place the mushrooms on a baking sheet greased with Pam.
2. Add pepper and salt to the mushrooms to taste and spray them with Pam.
3. Bake the mushrooms for 10-12 minutes.
4. Combine the following in a medium sized food bowl: leek, Worcestershire sauce, ground flax seeds, egg white, pepper, salt, garlic and onion powder.
5. Add in the finely chopped cooked shrimp and mix.
6. Divide the mixture into two.
7. Cook the patties on a skilled with Pam for 5-6 minutes. Flip over and cook the other side for the same duration.
8. Put 2-3 tablespoons of cottage cheese into a mushroom, the patties and the other mushroom cap on the top. Perform this with the other pair of mushroom caps, patties and cheese.

9. Place in the oven for 6-7 minutes to melt the cheese.
10. Serve and enjoy.

Hot Stir Fry a la Mexicana

The peppers in this recipe will boost your metabolism and will add some heat and variety to your diet.

Ingredients:

1 large tomato (diced)
1 large onion
1 Jalapeño pepper (minced)
3 skinless, boneless 150g chicken breasts, cut into cubes
3 medium red bell peppers, diced
Salt and pepper (to taste)
2 Serrano peppers (minced)
3 tablespoon chili powder

Here's how:

1. Put the skillet into medium flame and spray it with Pam.
2. Add in the chicken, salt, pepper and a tablespoon of chili powder.
3. Cook the chicken until it turns from pink to brown.
4. Set the chicken aside.
5. Using the same skillet, add in the peppers and onion and sauté.
6. Add in the tomato, chili powder (2 tablespoons), Jalapeño and Serrano's and stir fry the vegetables for 3-4 minutes.
7. Add in the chicken prepared in 3 and stir fry for another 3 more minutes.
8. Serve and enjoy.

Vegetable Mix à la Afrique

Ingredients:

3 tablespoon lemon juice (freshly squeezed)
2 teaspoon ground cumin
1/3 c fresh cilantro
15 oz. canned chickpeas (drained)
30 oz. canned diced tomatoes

1 tablespoon fresh ginger (grated)
2 bay leaves
1 large onion (cut in strips)
2lb cauliflower florets (cut into 2-inch pieces)
5 cloves of garlic (minced)
1 large zucchini (cut into 1-inch pieces)
1 teaspoon hot paprika
1 tablespoon cinnamon
½ teaspoon turmeric

Here's how:

1. Sauté onion in a large pan sprayed with Pam until it turns translucent.
2. Add in the ginger, gay leaves, lemon juice, salt, pepper, cumin, and paprika and cook them until soft.
3. Add in the cauliflower, tomatoes (including their juices), cinnamon and chickpeas with 2 cups of water and bring to boil.
4. Reduce the heat and simmer for 15-20 minutes. Stir it every 5 minutes.
5. Add the zucchini and cook until the zucchini is soft (usually around 10-12 minutes)
6. Remove from heat and serve. Enjoy.

Zero-Carb Lasagna

Ingredients:

1 lb zucchini, thinly sliced
1 large onion, chopped
1 teaspoon dried oregano
2 c broccoli florets, steamed and chopped
3 cloves of garlic, minced
2 egg whites
1 c fat free low sodium cottage cheese
1 teaspoon dried thyme
1 teaspoon dried rosemary
1 lb of extra lean ground turkey
1 c fat free sour cream
1 can of crushed tomatoes
1 teaspoon dried sage
2 c chopped spinach

Here's how:

1. Preheat the oven to about 375.
2. Spray Pam to a cooking pan and cook the meat until brown. Drain it and put it aside afterwards.
3. Using the same pan, sauté garlic and onion until the garlic turns golden.
4. Add in the meat, tomatoes, spinach and the seasonings.
5. In a medium sized food bowl, combine the egg whites, broccoli, salt, pepper and sour cream.
6. Placed the zucchini slices in the baking dish as the bottom layer.
7. Top it with half of the sour cream sauce and have the meat sauce.
8. Top it again with zucchini slices and use the remainder of the sour cream and meat sauce to top the second layer of zucchini slices.
9. Spread the cottage cheese on the top.
10. Cover the preparation with tin foil.
11. Bake it for 50 minutes to an hour.
12. Remove the tin foil covering and bake for another 10-15 minutes.
13. Cool and serve.

ChocoMocha Protein Mix

Ingredients:

½ scoops chocolate whey protein powder
1-2 cups ice cubes
1 cup non sweetened Almond Milk (Vanilla or Chocolate)
½ teaspoon cocoa powder
½ cup nonfat yogurt
1 teaspoon instant coffee (Nestle Vanilla or Hazelnut flavor is the best!)
2 packets stevia

Here's how:

1. Mix all the ingredients to a blender and process for 30 minutes to a full minute.

2. Serve and enjoy.

Almond Milk (Homemade)

Ingredients:

3 liters Spring water
Stevia (or any sweetener you prefer)
2 cups raw almonds

Here's how:

1. Soak the almonds overnight.
2. Blend 1 cup of almonds with three cups of water.
3. Add in your favorite sweetener and process.
4. Using a straining bag or a cheesecloth, strain the mixture into a pitcher (or bottle)
5. Repeat the process.

Chapter 5 – Grocery Shopping Tips For Atkins

It is important to realize that the market, which is the primary place for food, is filled with processed foods that contain carbohydrates that are easily converted into glucose and are converted to energy. Even those which seems to be low in carbohydrates or those which does not seem to have carbohydrates in their ingredients have hidden carbs that Atkins shopper must be wary of. Here are some tips to be a wise Atkins shopper:

- **Plan ahead.** The worst thing any shopper could do is to head on to the grocery store without a list of what to buy. A person could risk buying stuffs that he doesn't really need (or worse, foods that are not allowed in Atkins. Create a meal plan and base your list on the said plan. Go over the list of the ingredients needed to prepare the food included in your plan and check for carbohydrate sources in case one or two have been included.
- **Buy your proteins and produce first.** You don't have to think about the quality of the protein in meat so you don't need that much of a time selecting those. Once you have filled your cart with your produce and your proteins, you will have to hesitate about buying other stuff that are necessary or those which are just indulgence.
- **Buy meat in bulk.** Protein is the most important part of the Atkins and will replace most of your calories from carbohydrates while your body is transitioning to ketosis. Buying meat in bulk could also afford a person discounts. Also, having meat readily available could make planning and preparing meals for the week a lot easier.
- **Purchase cheese in bulk.** A lot of brand cheeses are offered in bulk and are cheaper compared to retailed ones. Ensure, however, that when you indulge in

cheese, you also eat food stuffs that are rich in fiber such as raw vegetables and salads.

- **Read labels and compare.** There is no better way at determining the nutritional contents and the composition of the food than the label. The label will tell how much salt, carbohydrate, sugar and fats are in the food. It also tells of what kind of fat are present in the food. Read labels and compare two products. As you continue to do the same routine, you will gradually build a list of the best food and which will make your grocery experience in the future a lot easier.
- **Take time.** Remember, Atkins diet is more than just a diet. It is a lifestyle. Part the lifestyle changes that you would have to embrace in order to fully benefit from the Atkins diet it to mind the quality and the quantity of the food that you eat.

Chapter 6 – How To Go Out To Eat On The Atkins Diet

It is ironic that one of the most potent threats to any form of weight loss diet or program is the very thing that medical experts prescribe: self-control.

Although, in essence, self-control is the key to discipline which ultimately leads to weight loss, reliance on it is not. Hunger and craving for food are genetically hardwired to every creature through millions of years of evolution. Your eight-day old decision to lose weight, which fuels your self-control, is not enough to counter that.

Here are some advices to keep your eye on the Atkins prize:

- **Gorge on salads first.** The idea is simple: stuff yourself with foods that are low in carbohydrates and filled with fiber first to have less space for other foods later. Fiber is the key component here as it slows down the digestion of carbohydrates particularly those which you may fail to detect.
- **Carry your own sauces, salad dressings and spices.** You won't get wrong with something you have prepared yourself. You can get an old multivitamin bottle and fill it with your homemade dressings.
- **Be prepared.** Observe your eating habits and remember what types of food or ingredients cause you to crave for carbohydrates and avoid the occasion of being exposed to those by requesting that you be served with alternatives.
- **Ask for alternatives.** Make it a habit to ask for substitutes for common high-carb ingredients in food and politely request to have your food be prepared the way you want.
- **Conquer the multitude of fast-food temptations.** Although it is best to avoid situations where you will be given a chance to stand long enough to be tempted near a fast food chain, the best way, still, is to bravely and intelligently confront fast food temptations right on its

face. There are fast foods that offer alternatives such as a Caesar side salad for French fries or a double burger without bun. Remember: you are only advised to cut on carbohydrates. These fast food restaurants have high-protein high-fat foods, too. Turn your mind to those.

- **Keep yourself well-hydrated.** Thirst can sometimes be mistaken for hunger which is a precursor for craving. The ideal water intake is 8 8-ounce glass of water a day. Atkins also cause to body to enter a state of ketosis which favors the abundant release of ketone bodies in the blood. Excess ketone bodies which are not used for energy are filtered through the kidneys. Without sufficient hydration, your kidneys will be overburdened.

Chapter 7 - Top Foods To Eat And Foods To Avoid

The success of Atkins diet greatly depends on the type of food you ingest. Here is the list of foods that should be included in the protein diet.

Foods to eat:

- **Meat.** The success of Atkin's diet can best be attributed its being a protein-heavy diet. Not only is protein a better substitute for Carbohydrates as an energy source, it is also instrumental in regulating one's appetite. As your body adjusts to a low-carb diet and as it transitions to ketosis, it will seek another source of energy. At the initial phase of the diet where your body is deprived of carbohydrates, it will not readily resort to utilizing fats as energy source. Instead, it will turn more to protein. Without sufficient supply of protein, your body will begin degrading your muscles in order to obtain protein for energy. This is counter by including a sufficient amount of protein in the diet—enough to supply your body's protein needs. Meat good for Atkins are bacon, pork, ham, beef, venison, veal and lamb. Be very careful when selecting your meat, though. Some processed meats, specially bacon and ham, are cured with sugar. This will not only add in to your carbohydrate consumptions but you might not even notice it. This result to your excess consumption of carbohydrates way past your daily allocation limit.
- **Eggs and poultry.** Poultry and eggs are also best sources of protein not only because of their being readily consumable or requiring less time to prepare but also because they are good sources of other nutrients that cannot be derived from most protein sources such as meat. Among these nutrients are beta-carotene, lutein, omega-3 and calcium. Among the best poultry foods and egg dishes that could be included in an Atkins diet are poached egg, soft and hard boiled

eggs, omelets, fried and scrambled eggs, deviled eggs, chicken, duck, pheasant, quail, goose, ostrich, turkey and Cornish hen.

- **Shellfish.** The best thing about non-restrictive diet, such as Atkins diet is that a dieter is not limited to a certain daily caloric requirement which could leave a dieter hungry. Those who are on Atkins diet could consume food as much as they want as long as the food is included in the list of allowed foods. Fortunately for Atkins, most delectable foods and dishes are not prohibited such as shellfish. Among the shellfish foods are squid, lobster, shrimp, mussels, crabmeat, clams and oysters.

- **Fish.** Fishes are excellent protein sources in Atkins diet as they contain healthy fats that may bolster the cardiovascular benefits of Atkins diet. Although studies and experiments comparing the effects of bad and good fats revealed both to have positive effect on cardiovascular health of a person with bad fats producing no bad effects, good fats from fish, still, have good effects which render them somewhat superior to meat. Among the fishes that are allowed to be included in this diet are flounder, salmon, sardines, herring, tuna, trout, halibut, and cod.

- **Cheese.** Cheeses adds flavor to food and makes your Atkins experience a lot better. Among the cheeses that could be eaten are blue cheeses, cream cheese, cheddar cheese, Gouda cheese, feta cheese, mozzarella, Swiss, and parmesan.

- **Vegetables.** One of the drawbacks of Atkins diet is its being low on fiber which makes most dieters constipated. In order to counter this, one must consume a liberal amount of vegetables. Because of restrictions in the amount of carbohydrates, however, one couldn't just eat any vegetable because some contains starch and carbohydrates sufficient enough to make a person's carbohydrate consumption past his limits. Vegetables that are allowed are alfalfa sprouts (1/2 cup/day and preferably raw), chives (1 tbsp./day), cucumber (1/2 cup/day), celery (1 stalk/day), chicory greens (1/2 cup/ day; preferably raw), bok choy (1 cup/day; preferably raw), peppers (1/2 cup/day;

preferably raw), radishes (6/day; preferably raw), romaine lettuce (1 cup/day; preferably raw), kohlrabi (1/4 cup/day), kale (1/2 cup/day), green strings of beans (1 cup/day).

- **Fats and oils.** The fuel of ketosis is fats and Atkins will not succeed without including fats in the diet. Essentially, Atkins does not provide any provisions on what kind of fats to include in the diet as ketosis renders all fat somewhat equal. Fats that should be included in your diet are: Canola, soybean, grape seed, sesame, sunflower, safflower, and walnut.
- **Sweeteners.** Atkins does not favor restrictions in the amount of food or the enjoyment a dieter feels as this can lead to hunger and craving. It does not even favor that the quality of food be compromised due to avoidance of carbohydrates. To make your eating experience more worthwhile, you can use sweeteners. The best sweetener for Atkins diet is Splenda.
- **Drinks and beverages.** Drinks for Atkins include herb tea, diet soda, cream, club soda, clear broth, unflavored soy/almond milk and water.

Foods to Avoid Atkins

There are foods that seem healthy but are actually detrimental in Atkins. Those are foods that have hidden carbohydrates in them which could prevent ketosis. These are:

- **Milk substitutes.** Although soy and almond milks lack lactose, a form of sugar and a carbohydrate source, be very wary of the flavored ones. A cup of vanilla almond milk, for example, has 16 g of carbohydrates and a cup of chocolate soy milk has 23 grams of carbohydrates compared to unflavored soy milk.
- **Yoghurt.** Although yoghurt is a good source of dietary calcium and of probiotics (organisms which help keep a healthy intestinal environment), it is better to avoid eating one during the Induction Phase of Atkins as a regular low-fat one contains as much as 40 grams of carbohydrates. Even the Greek yogurt version packs a

whopping 9g rams of carb—enough to fill half of your carbohydrate requirement for the day.

- **Tomato Sauce.** It its over-the-counter, ready-made
- **Beans.** Even a cup of baked beans contain 54 grams of carbohydrates from its starch contents. If you enjoy beans, you can either include it at the second part of your diet as you go along carbohydrate intake increments or limit your consumption to an amount that could give you 20 g of carb a day.

Chapter 8 - Health Benefits Of The Atkins Diet

Experts agree that large amounts of carbohydrates were not originally part of the usual human diet and that the homeostatic condition of the human body is not optimized for a high-carbohydrate diet.

The introduction of refined carbohydrates as alternative and modern sources of calories was so abrupt that the human body has had no chance of adapting. This explains why so many people nowadays are having difficulty losing and maintaining weight.

Reverting to a low-carbohydrate diet, such as the Atkins diet, has been proven to be beneficial to health. Among the benefits are:

- **Weight loss.** Not only is excess weight associated with cardiovascular diseases and diabetes, carrying an extra weight adds strain to joints and body parts that may cause other health problems such as joint pains, bone fracture and bruises, among others. The first noticeable health benefit of an Atkins diet is nothing more than losing the pesky extra pounds itself.
- **Blood sugar normalized.** While at Atkins, the body does not need insulin in order to keep blood sugar at normal levels. Because of limited carbohydrates in diet, blood sugar levels in the blood remain low while still having ketones for energy source. People with problems in insulin sensitivity or with insulin production will particularly benefit from this type of diet.
- **Reduced triglyceride levels.** The amount of triglycerides in the blood determines the person's cardiovascular health. Blood concentration of more than 100 mg/dL increases a person's risk of heart attack, stroke and cardiovascular diseases. A study conducted by the Department of Medicine at the University of Western Ontario, London involving ten healthy subjects reveal an improvement in triglyceride levels in the blood following a high-fat high-protein

low-carbohydrate (Atkins) diet for four weeks. This only proves that Atkins diet is beneficial to maintaining a healthy cardiovascular system.

- **Increased HDL Cholesterol Levels.** A study conducted by Ronald Krauss and his colleagues reveal that high-fat, high-protein low-carbohydrate diet increases the persons HDL (good) level while decreasing LDL (bad) cholesterol levels even if the person under the diet exhibited no weight loss. Those who have lost weight on the diet have even exhibited further improvements in their HDL and LDL levels.
- **Blood pressure normalizes.** A research conducted in the General Clinical Research Centers of the Hospital and the Children's Hospital of Boston reveals that Atkins diet (and any diet low in carbohydrate) can help maintain a normal blood pressure and prevent the health risks associated with prolonged hypertension.

Chapter 9 – Avoiding Crucial Mistakes

Although perfectionism is not required in Atkins at it is so easy and dieter-friendly that one could easily keep up with the steps well without keeping much thought about it, there are still things that must be avoided in order to ensure the program's success. After all, one mistake could nullify even your months of effort. Here are the mistakes a dieter could commit and the ways to avoid them:

- **Counting the total instead of net carbohydrates.** Net carbs is defined as the difference between the total carbohydrates and fiber in grams. That is, in order to determine the net carbohydrate content of food, you need to subtract the amount of fiber to the amount of carbohydrates of food. Another way of ensuring that you stay with the prescribed carbohydrate allowance is to count each sugar substitute you use on food (as sweetener) as 1 g of net carbohydrates.
- **Eating fewer vegetables.** A rule of thumb to not go wrong here is to acquire your net carb requirement for the day from vegetables. Vegetables are the best sources of carbohydrates because of their fiber content and the other nutrients they contain. Experts advise to eat as much as 6 cups of green leafy vegetables and 2 cubs of cooked vegetables a day.
- **Not keeping yourself hydrated enough.** While Atkins allows your body to speed up your fat metabolism through decreased carbohydrate intake, the production of ketone bodies associated with fat metabolism overwhelms the kidneys. Without much hydration, the kidneys will have difficulty filtering out excess ketones and other waste products from the blood. In worst cases, stones could even form. This is countered by drinking at lease 8 8-ounce glass of water a day.
- **Insufficient protein intake.** It has been demonstrated that low-carbohydrate diet, when done incorrectly, could result to your body using your protein reserves from muscles for energy instead of your adipose

deposits. In order to prevent this, Atkins dieters should consume sufficient amounts of protein to initiate protein sparing. This translates to as much as 4-6 ounces of protein per meal.

- **Avoiding salt.** During the induction phase, much electrolyte is lost during the initial and rapid water-weight loss. This can result to weakness, headaches, muscle cramps, vertigo and various discomforts. A sufficient amount of salt on the diet could provide the necessary electrolytes and diminish or avoid these effects.
- **Not eating fat.** Being afraid of fat is normal as experts have been convincing people, out of honest belief, that fats are bad. The major source of energy in the Atkins diet, though, is no longer glucose but ketones derived from fats. Not ingesting enough fat could cause your body to use your fat reserves at a pace that is no longer comfortable for your body.
- **Hidden carbs.** It is crucial that a person stick to the prescribed carbohydrate intake all throughout the duration of Atkins in order to sustain ketosis. Not accounting hidden carbs could render all your dieting efforts futile. It can also be detrimental as there are cases where people who have undergone a failed and fluctuating ketosis exhibit increase insulin sensitivity which leads to insulin resistance later on.

Chapter 10 - Staying Motivated

Compared to other diets, low-carbohydrate diets are more likely to be continued for longer periods of time even after a dieter has achieved his desired weight. This is because Atkins does not cause hunger or deprivation and craving and is shown to reduce a person's appetite over time. Nevertheless, there are still people who would break out of ketosis and of Atkins diet because of poor motivation despite excellent results. Here are some steps to ensure that you keep motivated with the Atkins diet.

- **Be positive.** As with all endeavors, the key to perseverance is optimism and the desire to achieve positive results. You can adapt a mantra and repeat it to yourself every morning. Some even write their mantras on a piece of paper and stick it to their mirrors. Positive mantras may not seem to do an effect but experts found out that this activity, which is a form of self-motivation, subconsciously cause a persons' behavior to change in order to follow the mantra.
- **Plan your meals and stick to it.** If you have problem with self-control and focus, you can write your meals down for the day (or the week) and prepare them yourself. Doing this will remove the necessity to fight temptation and will increase the likelihood of you focusing and consuming only the foods that are part of the diet.
- **Divide the whole process into small achievable goals.** One of the most effective zappers of motivation is the lack of feeling of achievement. This has nothing to do with whether a person actually achieves something or not but has more to do with how he perceives and appreciates the outcome. One of the ways to help you with your focus is to feed yourself constantly with the feeling and sense of achievement by setting smaller goals. You can increase the feeling of achievement by giving yourself a reward afterwards.
- **Don't frequently check for stats.** Although it may be a good way to check your progress, checking for your stats often, though, will decrease your motivation. This

is because the more frequent you check, the more you would expect to see changes. As with most diets which start the weight loss off rapidly, checking for your stats after this initial rapid weight loss would cause disappointment as the succeeding weight loss is expected to occur at a significantly slower pace.

- **Enlist the support of your family.** Sometimes, internal motivation is just not enough. Enlisting the help of family and friends could encourage us to stay motivated further because we tend to listen to what other people say specially those of a group of people.

Over-all, though, years of testimonies and results reveal that Atkins is not difficult to maintain. In fact, a significant number of people have adapted Atkins as a way of life for years now and have benefited greatly from the array of its health effects.

Conclusion

Thank you again for purchasing this book on *Ultimate Atkins Diet Quick Start Tool Kit!*!

I am extremely excited to pass this information along to you, and I am so happy that you now have read and can hopefully implement these strategies going forward.

I hope this book was able to help you understand Atkins diet, the processes involved in ketosis and the ways on how to benefit from either this diet or this state of increased fat metabolism

The next step is to get started using this information and to hopefully live a fuller, energy-filled life without the need for counting calories or being conscious of your body shape and size!

Please don't be someone who just reads this information and doesn't apply it, the strategies in this book will only benefit you if you use them!

If you know of anyone else that could benefit from the information presented here please inform them of this book.

Finally, if you enjoyed this book and feel it has added value to your life in any way, please take the time to share your thoughts and post a review on Amazon. It'd be greatly appreciated!

Thank you and good luck!

Preview Of:

<u>Low Carb Diet</u>

Low Carb Diet Plan For Fat Loss For Life! Fast Acting Low Carb Diet To Lose Weight As Soon As Tomorrow!

Introduction

I want to thank you and congratulate you for purchasing the book, *"Low Carb Diet: Low Carb Diet Plan For Fat Loss For Life! Fast Acting Low Carb Diet To Lose Weight As Soon As Tomorrow!"*.

This book contains proven steps and strategies on how to get rid of excess weight fast!

So you have found yourself in the position of procrastination. You needed to start dieting months ago to get ready for that special event, or just to get ready to go to the beach or pool this year. Don't dismay you are not alone or too late. There are many proven strategies that can help you lose those extra pounds.

If you need to lose 10 lbs fast, drop a few inches to fit into that dress or maybe to fit into those favorite pants once again, then this book is exactly what you need. It will provide you with all the latest techniques and strategies to give you the surefire way to accomplish your desires in record time.

Don't wait any longer to have the body and health you have been missing out on. Many people wait for a perfect time to get in shape, lose a few pounds, and feel better about themselves, only to lose precious years in the process. The problem is that many times there isn't a perfect time to do anything in our lives.

The perfect time is NOW. If you really want something, there is no such thing as the wrong timing. Just take action now and you will soon be on your way to a much happier life.

Thanks again for purchasing this book, I hope you enjoy it!

Chapter 1: Faster Low Carb Weight Loss Strategies

One of the most common physical problems in our modern world is people gaining unwanted fat in problem areas of their body's. The easy availability of cheap fast food and other unhealthy processed food have caused people to lose control of their diet. After looking in the mirror and realizing how much they have gained, people often are left with feelings of sadness, discouragement, and wondering if their long term health is at risk.

The great Tony Robbins says that we need to see our problems as they are, but not worse than they are. So let us take his advice and realize all we need to do is change a few things in our diet, exercise program, and begin living a healthier lifestyle to fix our seemingly large problems that in reality are not that hard to fix! So let's not overcomplicate them.

Slimming down does not necessarily mean you have to starve yourself. Provided the right diet and a proper exercise plan, it is not impossible to lose 10 pounds fast. So what does it exactly take to slim down fast enough? Below are some of the most important things you should keep in mind:

- Make complex carbs 30 percent of you calorie consumption

- Make protein 50 percent of your calorie intake

- Make healthy fats 20 percent of the total calories you eat

Avoid the common weight loss mistakes.

When it comes to losing the extra pounds, it is not only important that you learn the things you should be doing. It is equally crucial that you figure out the wrong things you may still be doing. A lot of people do weight loss mistakes without even knowing it. Little do they know what they think can slim them down are actually obstacles to their weight loss goals.

For instance, skipping meals is one of the most common practices. The plain truth is that it is an unhealthy practice. Some people also avoid dairy products altogether. But the fact is calcium contained in dairy products is helpful in burning calories and fat.

Water should not be avoided when dieting. Water can not only burn fat, it also helps the body get rid of toxins. Ice cold water for instance is very good because the body is forced to burn additional calories and fat to make sure the water you drink is properly heated to match your body temperature. You are also more than welcome to dose up on coconut water, fat free milk and other slimming drinks such as green tea, vegetable juice and yogurt based smoothies.

Stick to a healthy diet plan.

You have plenty of food options to include in your diet. The safest bet always includes raw fruits and vegetables. These healthy foods work not only to slim you down but also promote your overall health. These foods also give you energy to perform slimming exercises which can only increase the amount of weight loss.

Sufficient amount of fruits and vegetables included regularly in your daily meals ensures that you are getting enough fiber from your diet. Fibers are known to be good for digestion and assist in gradual weight loss. Fruits are a little tricky because they do have higher sugar content, so you will want to make sure you get a serving or two, but also make sure that they don't push you over the edge in the way of your low-carb diet guidelines.

Vegetables on the other hand, are pretty hard to eat too many of, especially the green kind. Think spinach leaves, broccoli, kale, cucumbers, zucchini squash, etc...When you veer off into the colored ones like carrots just make sure you know what is in them, because carrots for instance actually have quite a bit of sugar! This doesn't mean they can't be eaten or that they shouldn't be, it just means moderation is probably a good idea.

Make time for exercise.

Dieting alone will not suffice. Cardiovascular exercises are recommended for overall weight loss. But there are targeted forms of workout too. Know your goal and implement the right type of exercise including the proper equipment for best results.

People tend to avoid exercise thinking that a strict low-carb diet alone can help them get slim. Although true to some extent, it is very difficult to maintain proper weight loss without engaging in suitable exercises from time to time. Doing even light exercises is also effective if done correctly.

Why low-carb diet?

The advantage of a low carb diet over a low calorie diet is that a low-carb diet does not mean eating less food. It just means consuming less carbohydrates and sugar. Even foods having good quantities of fats are acceptable in a low carbohydrate diet plan, and in fact you should eat more healthy fats on a low carb diet to make sure you get the proper amount of calories - but I must stress this - fats add up quick! Be careful, a small handful of nuts, or half an avocado has a lot more calories than you think!

Low carb diets are known to help lose weight and also control blood-sugar level altogether without starving oneself.

The reason low-calorie diet is more popular is that, people think it shows faster and better results. But it also requires plenty of exercise for quick fat loss. Many people think they do not have adequate time for such routines. But I promise you there is time, it doesn't matter how many hours you work, or what your schedule, if you don't make time for your health, it will make time for you! And then it will be an emergency instead of a want.

Many of the world's leading physicians suggest low carb diet to their clients and get better results.

Although the main purpose of this type of diet is to lower carbohydrate intake, it is also important to know that long term deprivation of carbs in your body could damage your metabolism and decreases your fat burning capacity. So it is suggested that a limited but sufficient amount of carbohydrate intake is necessary daily. Also, this is why it is very important to have a higher carb day about one day a week, often called a cheat meal or day. When you do this you must abstain from over eating, this is not a high calorie day, just a high carb day, so this means that when you increase you carbs, you must lower your fats substantially to stay within your calorie range.

It is observed that low-carb diets also show similar outcomes as compared to low-calorie diet, with much less stress on our body. But you still have to manage your diet properly and adjust your eating and drinking habits accordingly.

Keep yourself away from stress. Being stressed gets your body in a state with elevated levels of stress related hormones. Increased stress actually increases your cravings for unhealthier food. This is not good for your low carb diet. If you are unsure of how this can be accomplished, I recommend checking out a book on meditation.

This all means you have to be ready to make changes on your lifestyle. A few sacrifices and compromises are called for here and there, but you know it is worth it when you start to get in a better shape.

Thanks for Previewing My Exciting Book Entitled:

"Low Carb Diet: Low Carb Diet Plan For Fat Loss For Life! Fast Acting Low Carb Diet To Lose Weight As Soon As Tomorrow!"

To purchase this book, simply go to the Amazon Kindle store and simply search:

' LOW CARB DIET"

Then just scroll down until you see my book. You will know it is mine because you will see my name "Sarah Brooks" underneath the title.

Alternatively, you can visit my author page on Amazon to see this book and other work I have done. Thanks so much, and please don't forget your free bonuses

DON'T LEAVE YET! - CHECK OUT YOUR FREE BONUSES BELOW!

Free Bonus Offer: Get Free Access To The www.LiveFitVIP.com VIP Newsletter!

Once you enter your email address you will immediately get free access to this awesome newsletter!

But wait, right now if you join now for free you will also get free access to the "The 7 Keys To Body Transformation" free EBook!

To claim both your FREE VIP NEWSLETTER MEMBERSHIP and your FREE BONUS Ebook on THE 7 KEYS TO BODY TRANSFORMATION!

Just Go To:

www.liveFitVIP.com